EXERCISES FOR BAD POSTURE

EVERYTHING YOU NEED TO IMPROVE POSTURE IN JUST A FEW MINUTES PER DAY

ALIOS JOHNSON

Table of Contents

ABOUT THE AUTHOR

Alios has in his lifetime always been a huge fan of optimizing the human body to function at its best and most healthy state. In his daily life he helps a lot of people with physical therapy treatment in his own clinic based in the heart of New York. Inside his clinic he also helps people with improving mental health. That includes stress management, anxiety, anger, eating disorders, sleep problems and much more. In his spare time he enjoys writing about all aspects of health and fitness, so that he can reach people all over the world and leave an impression that may even change some lives out there. He does personal training also, delivering value to a handful of clients to achieve their fitness goals.

Besides his passion for helping others, Alios also loves to keep himself as healthy as possible, which is why he has dedicated his life to physical exercise, yoga, meditation, posture correction and many other healthy activities.

INTRODUCTION

Posture may be termed as good or bad and is often relevant to good and bad postural habits. Posture may be defined as the ability to maintain the upright position against the force of gravity so that it prevents one falling over. However, posture is also involved in sitting, lying, stooping, squatting as well as being erect. Habits are learned responses to the environment. The tall teenager, for example may develop rounded shoulders in the attempt to blend in with his/her peers instead of towering above them. It takes time to acquire a habit but once the habit is installed in the subconscious mind, it is difficult to shift.

Good posture suggests a balance and alignment between the muscular and skeletal structures, protecting our bodies from injury and degenerative changes. Muscles, ligaments, tendons, fascia and bony skeleton work together to keep us moving, sitting, standing, and lying down at our request. We have a whole team at our disposal waiting for instructions from above to set us into motion. Our muscular-skeletal system gives us shape, helping to keep the internal organs in place. A well-balanced body is one that feels energetic while a poorly balanced system often feels languid, generally out of sorts and less able to cope with the demands of everyday life. It often has less stamina and can be easily overwhelmed, which has the potential to lead to melt down (burn out). This in turn can affect the hormonal system.

Working arrangements. How we sit or stand and for how long. What type of work do you do? Is it sedentary or heavy, physical work? What is the temperature like? Hot, cold, air-conditioned, draughty conditions can affect the way we react to our environment. Is our work repetitive and maybe we use telephone, computer, carry shopping or schoolbags, laptops etc. Are we fit enough for the job and do we drink enough water during the day? Is our work stressful or does it make us tense and reactive to everyday situations? Constant deadlines, too much caffeine, driving, carrying a heavy handbag on one shoulder are some of the examples that can change us from that lovable, charming individual to a screaming, out of control colleague that is frankly best avoided.

Imagine a line dropped from the middle of your ear down through the middle of your shoulder to the centre of your ankle. Does yours do that? Try checking it in a mirror. Our Victorian ancestors were sticklers for good posture. True for the ladies, at least, it may have something to do with their whalebone corsets, which were often pulled far too tight for any sort of comfort. The Victorians liked to sit ramrod straight often on very hard chairs.

Today's society views matter differently. We tend to be more relaxed about posture and yet someone who carries themself well often comes across as someone with confidence. If you are going for a job interview, your posture is often far more important than the clothes you are wearing. If you stand or sit upright, clothes look so much better and so too does the impression that you are creating. While looks play an important role, faulty posture has the potential to lead to pain and discomfort, which if ignored for long enough may lead to degenerative changes and disability. Mention the word posture and for many people they simply try to sit up straight but without a properly balanced underlying structure, it is often very difficult to maintain. The brain has become used to instructing the body to move in a certain manner and it will resist change. Change is frightening and is something that people find hard to embrace. A case of the mind is willing but the flesh is weak.

There are therapies available to help you make the most of your own personal resources. Bowen is one that particularly excels with rebalancing the muscular skeletal structures. It does it in a totally non-threatening way and works with the mind-body relationship as well as the structural entity. It is thought that the mind controls 80% of the body's health with the remaining 20% often emerging as a physical manifestation of, for example, pain. Whilst a single treatment can go a long way in the task of re-educating the working capability of the body, it generally requires a course of treatment to set it on the right track with a maintenance programme of usually a single follow-up treatment at regular intervals. The interval varies from individual to individual.

You may be wondering is it really that simple? Can this be true? The body likes to be in balance. It functions much more efficiently and has more energy. In other words, you feel better. Even if your posture is not the greatest in the world, there are in many cases, great improvements to be made. With more energy, there are more resources to do more and to be more. There are fewer tendencies to injury and to maximize results. Net outcome happiness and fulfilment and for many people this is exactly what they want. Remember with a little help the body has its own resources to correct many postural deficiencies. Why don't you give it a try and find out for yourselves?

THE IMPORTANCE OF GOOD POSTURE AND AGING

Practically every part of the body deteriorates at some point in time. It is all a part of the aging process that is inevitable for everyone regardless of their stature in life. Carrying or lifting things now becomes a conscious effort, even simple chores like climbing up the stairs or sitting can be daunting.

What Happens To Our Body When We Age?

By the time you reach your 50s or 60s, you will probably notice something peculiar. You might observe half an inch or one-inch difference in your height. This is a natural process brought about by the shrinking of your spine.

Your spine is made up of vertebrae and between them are discs that serve as a cushion. As time goes by, these discs lose their form and begin to thin down. Add to that, your cartilage and connective tissues lose thickness and elasticity. All these things might not be cosmetically noticeable at first. However, this could have been prevented if we exhibit good harmony to our body through proper posture, healthy eating, and regular exercise.

Posture is one thing not everyone takes seriously, but it is very important as it promotes independent lifestyle and movement. Having proper posture improves your balance and symmetry. It can prevent you from having hunched shoulders, back pains, and shrinking spine. In part, it also makes you look good and feel good. All in all, having good posture is a good indicator of how well you will age later on in your life.

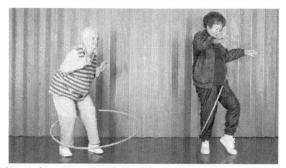

What Are The Advantages of Good Posture To Seniors?

There are many health problems brought about by poor posture, and correcting the habit can go a long way. Nonetheless, good posture has to start somewhere. The perfect place is the spine. Few know that our spine carries about 10 pounds of weight everyday. Once you hunch forward, gravity pulls it further causing the spine to tighten. A series of consequences follows after.

For one, this can be the cause of headaches. As you hunch forward when sitting, tension in the cervical vertebrae is built up, causing it to be out of alignment. And over time, misalignment causes blood vessels to be pinched, limiting their capability to supply blood to the brain, which later promotes migraines and headaches.

Poor posture can lead to back pain. As you slouch, the muscles and ligaments in your back struggle and are pressured to maintain your balance. Pulling the muscles, especially in the lumbar area where most weight is carried, causes back pain. Over time, this habit can cause fast degeneration of the spine, which can lead to serious complications like osteoarthritis, scoliosis, and osteoporosis.

Poor posture also compresses internal organs, decreasing their functionality and efficiency. Studies also show that slouching has a major effect to digestion and blood flow. Because of this, seniors can develop hypertension or low metabolic rate, and put them at risk of heart attack, stroke, and even diabetes and obesity. Add to this, hunching the back makes the rib cage constricted, leaving the lungs as well as the heart limited space to function well. More so, too much pressure put on the spine can press important blood vessels, limiting proper blood flow, which is essential for nourishing and originating these vital organs.

Now that we know how our bad posture habits can cause tremendous health risks to our body, making a conscious effort to change this through posture exercise training can turn the tables. Through proper posture, seniors may no longer experience chest pains, back aches, headaches, and will have better digestion. And if you are still not convinced, further benefits of good posture affect a senior's state of mind. It has been proven that sitting or standing upright can promote positivity, which gives more confidence to our own thoughts and decision making.

In an experiment, having good posture showed that seniors developed better memory recall. Although this is not yet proof that proper posture can slow down the process of Alzheimer's, having the spine properly aligned while standing or sitting makes neurotransmitters communicate faster from the brain to every part of the body, making it easy to retain memory.

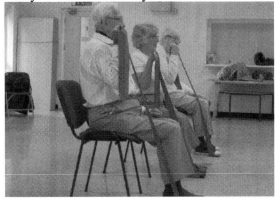

Good posture can also eliminate depression. By sitting and walking straight, energy levels are boosted. People with poor posture are prone to panic, anxiety, and shallow breathing, making it hard to overcome negativity. Good posture improves circulation, oxygenating the body well, and boosting perception and thinking, leaving one more at peace and ready to face any problem that may come the senior's way. Getting involved in an elderly exercise program is a good way to start.

Indeed, for seniors to start thinking about their posture early on can help them grace their way through the aging process. And if proper posture is complemented with regular exercise and healthy diet, aging for any senior will just be another phase that they can enjoy more and benefit from.

THE SENSATION OF GOOD POSTURE

The sensation of good posture is very pleasurable. Those with good posture are using the appropriate muscles for movement and stability. These people feel free and easy, at least in their physical movements, and very likely in how they feel about themselves. They walk gracefully and look as though they know that they have that certain "something." They easily engage with others having the same easy sensation. People within this group of posture perfect individuals are exchanging glances, rewarding smiles, and pleasant discussions. These are empowering social exchanges that lift their spirits for their whole day, the whole week, and throughout their lives.

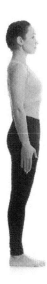

People with good posture showcase how they feel. They have a sense of communication above what is understood by those without good posture. They use their body language to send messages to each other.

These messages are actually what may be referred to as "vibes." These vibes or positive feelings transfer almost instantaneously to their electrical/chemical impulses. In fact these feelings are their impulses.

There is no need to be left out of this group of people. We all have electrical/chemical impulses that initiate our emotions and our physical muscle movements as a "reaction." (These impulses are also self triggered, however in this discussion let's review those impulses triggered by others who react toward us.) This meeting on the street for example, actually is an exchange of positive electrical/chemical reactions. If you have the right stuff, then you are appreciated when you are viewed. When you receive positive communication, say a pleasant "hello," or a kind look, electrical/chemical reactions are felt within you and they are soothing and enjoyable. We'll get to just how you can naturally be part of this selective group of people. Let's discuss more of what this body language is and the associated sensations.

Most of the time our own emotional sensations originate within our soul, our personality. When we improve ourselves physically, then emotionally, we'll have the personality and upright way in our movements to display a sense of peace and kindness toward others. Our own body in turn feels a certain satisfaction derived from their kind response. We can then easily exhibit an even more uplifting body and facial appearance. That's just how it works.

It can work for us or against us. When people see our way of moving or our appearance, are they inspired? Do they like what they see? Do they feel comfortable so they can exchange pleasantries? These are important questions. Let's delve into this.

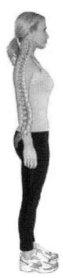

Think of communication as a two-way street or better, a cloverleaf on ramp to the "smooth highway" of socializing. There are many subtleties that one experiences as we communicate with others. To be rewarded with these pleasant sensations one must appear able to accept them. This is the two way street. Even a neutral but poised appearance on your part will bring about pleasant comments from others. The key for all this to happen often is to have the pleasing body posture and face that causes others to compliment you or at least notice you appreciably. This is the "smooth highway" mentioned earlier. The unspoken language of your body brings about a cause and effect when meeting others. Let's make it a positive and smooth cause and effect. Let's find out how we can do it.

How can you stimulate others to give you rewarding compliments? You can, of course, communicate with them verbally. This is important and useful. However if you have a posture that appears defeated or uninspired when talking, you may have an uphill battle to win the confidence and friendship of others.

What I wish to discuss with you in particular is the unspoken body language of good posture. A good posture is key when socializing. (a posture of grace and poise, not one of ramrod military bearing.) It is key when you make a first impression. It is key when you are viewed from afar. It is useful when you socialize because you are telling someone that you are comfortable, kind to yourself, kind to others. You are telling others that you can be trusted, you are easy to get along with and have what it takes to be associated with anyone. With good posture, you can begin to trust yourself so that you are able to choose good friends. You become more selective. Now you find that it is difficult to be friends with those who do not have similar good tastes as you. Your time and efforts won't be wasted on those who have tastes and traits that you find undesirable.

These are the many emotional and mental facets of socializing when you have good posture. I have yet to discuss physically how good it feels just to stand walk or sit properly or how our unburdened muscles "appreciate us" when we walk correctly. Our body's ease of movement rewards us. Our face becomes more relaxed and more prone to smiling. Our muscles become more streamlined, lengthened, and form a smooth base for the skin to layer upon. Our bones, comprised of 25% water, actually lengthen themselves to a small degree, as our lengthening muscles encourages them to do so. Our whole skeleton lengthens as we think "upwardly." Thus our skeletal framework is "open" to accept the continued growth of our muscles and our soft tissue, no matter what age or what physical state we may be in presently. We can change for the better.

Almost all of us have bodies that at birth, arrived with all the bones, nervous system, muscles, etc, to develop into a fine, normal human being. We have a body with all the implements to move about gracefully. We have miss used ourselves, or someone perhaps misguided us up to now, teaching us how to have bad posture. We now perhaps hurry to grab or do something, too quickly we walk with little coordination. This is called "end-gaining" and we focus too much upon reaching the end point of an objective. It is unfortunate that we do not permit ourselves to enjoy the "means-whereby" to get to a certain goal. Realizing this, it is entirely possible to change for the better by switching our focus from end-gaining to concentrating on the means-whereby. To begin a physical change simply lengthen the body. Doing this will help you mentally change for the better.

Lengthen your spine, free your neck and balance you head atop your shoulders will vastly improve your posture and appearance. In fact you owe it to yourself to better your appearance and posture. You must find a personal path to enjoy yourself and others by acquiring a better posture. You must find a way to move about with grace and poise, and to enjoy the sensations of ease of movement. The sensations and impulses you feel are what F.M Alexender says is our "inherent supremacy." When achieving such a graceful way of moving, one's body tells oneself that, "I am feeling more confident and I have a greater poise. I have more self-control over circumstances in my life. I feel a certain type of supremacy."

Sensations are something that you must feel personally. You must reclaim these personal feelings from those that you gave to others, even when you give them away to appropriate teachers. How can you allow another person to describe the sensations you'll feel? For example, what happens if you are asked by a teacher of the Alexander Technique to "turn you head at the very top of the spine, the C1 vertebra, and not with the neck at the C7 vertebra." Can the teacher describe the subtle sensations you feel? Somewhat but not fully. With due respect to the AT teachers, and I have much respect for those in this field, they may describe the feelings you achieve such as having a lighter walk or being more perceptive. In truth, sensations are difficult to describe. There would be too many words required, to many subjective thoughts to verbalize, so descriptions would be inadequate to state how you really feel. Sensations are difficult to describe. This sensation of lengthening the spine and balancing the head atop the spine must be felt by the person who is doing the changing for the better. You must allow yourself to personally enjoy these powerful uplifting feelings. Acquiring and enjoying such grace, poise and personal power is a yours alone to feel.

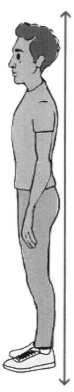

One must personally make the effort to change and enjoy these changes as you gain a better posture. One must personally feel the pleasant sensations of a graceful walk or stance. The best way of being "described" the sensation you may feel is not by a person of authority i.e. a teacher or an instructor. No, the best description, or feedback, of how you feel when improving your posture is when you are complimented. This can happen anywhere, anytime, which makes it all the more refreshing. It could be in a social setting, formal or informal, on the street, or in the office. This type of communication cuts through the technical jargon. Your senses note a real achievement of posture improvement when there is a pleasant interaction by your peers, acquaintances or someone new.

Above all, the very best person to describe, or sense, how you feel when you make a change for the better is you. You know when you have a lightened way of movement. You know what posture adjustment you made to become more graceful. You know what poise you've learned, and now exhibit, to make yourself more attractive and robust. Trust yourself. Once gaining a good posture and a certain poise, you are then prepared to like or love yourself more. You are prepared to accept complements. How one feels about themselves when offered kind comments is something to be felt or sensed, not something described to us.

So do all that you can to allow yourself to enjoy these moments when compliments are given to you. Whether these compliments are subtle glances your way, or the opposite sex moving into your personal space, a touch or a soft spoken word, they come in many forms. As simple as being asked over for dinner, or offered a drink of water can be considered a compliment. Doing all that you can to do to accept compliments includes improving posture, gaining grace and poise. When you improve your posture, compliments come in greater numbers. As your posture improves, so does your self-assurance, and so does your life.

Remember to passively exercise. By that I mean lengthen the spine, free the neck and align it with the more vertical spine. Balance the head a top the neck and above the lifted shoulders. Allow the sternocleidomastoid muscles (the front pair of neck muscles) to pull up the clavicles and sternum so the shoulders and chest rise. Loosen the jaw and breathe through the nose. Do this subtly. Do it for a better you. You will be appreciably regarded.

BAD POSTURE

We've been told time and time again to "sit up straight" or "stop slouching", but have we ever considered the health benefits of having good posture? In fact, people often attempt to fix their posture merely because it makes them look more confident, slimmer, and attractive. While all this may be true, bad posture can create many health issues that should be reason enough to work towards better posture. For example, bad posture is linked to chronic back pain, migraines, poor digestion, lack of oxygen flow, and much more.

Poor posture or "postural dysfunction" is defined as when our spine is being held in an unnatural position. The result of these unnatural positions are extra stress on our joints, muscles, and vertebrae. Most often, poor posture is something that we naturally do without even noticing. Anyone can suffer from poor posture and if you begin poor posture at a young age, is it likely you will carry it throughout your life. People are becoming more and more susceptible to posture issues because of the use of technology, forcing us to hold ourselves in unique positions to view a small screen. Unless you are actively working towards good posture, you are most likely making some type of posture mistake without even realizing it.

What are the Negative Effects of Poor Posture?

Poor posture has the potential to create numerous health issues including:

Low energy levels - The shallow breathing created by bad posture causes our energy levels to lower greatly.

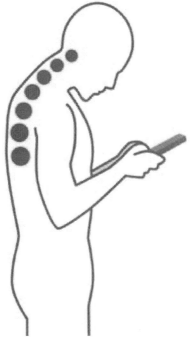

Chronic neck and back pain - Sitting or standing in slouched positions for any extended period of time puts extreme stress on your back and neck. At first this pain may just be short and acute. However, over time poor posture can do as much as completely misalign your spine.

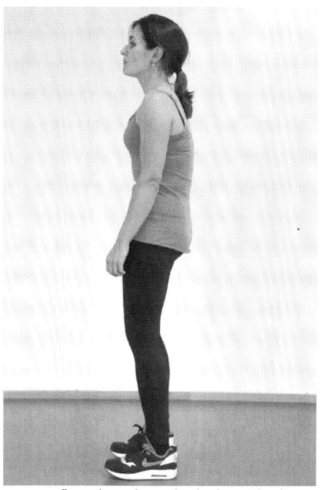

Lack of oxygen flow throughout the body - The lungs function correctly when the diaphragm and rib cage properly expand. In essence, having poor posture restricts blood and oxygen flow because the expansion isn't happening correctly.

Heart problems - The muscle strain and poor posture of the spine and rib cage negatively impact your heart health. This is mostly because of the lack of blood flow that occurs when you hunch over for extended periods of time. Also, any type of misalignment of your spine has the trickle down effect on other parts of your body.

Migraines and tension headaches - migraines and tension headaches are most commonly seen in people who spend all day working at a desk. The strain placed on the body from holding oneself incorrectly makes a person vulnerable to migraines and tension headaches. The lack of blood and oxygen flow to the head is also a component of this type of pain.

Lack of confidence - Many studies have shown a connection between someone who slouches and a lack of confidence. Often times these studies take it a step further saying that people who slouch are more likely to suffer from depression, stating people who slouch when they walk tend to experience increased feelings of depression and decrease levels of energy.

Digestion issues - Sitting for most of the day starts to constrict your intestines. The constriction of your intestines can make digestion a big problem. Poor posture has been attributed to issues like acid reflux and hernias.

Poor posture can come in a variety of different shapes and sizes. Everyone has their own way of incorrectly holding their posture. However, some posture issues are more common than others.

Problem: Slouching in a Chair
Many people have become accustomed to the chair slouch because sitting straight doesn't feel natural or comfortable. The natural tendency of a person sitting down for extended periods of time is to slouch over or down in the chair. This type of slouching is especially common with kids, teens, and people who work sedentary jobs. Over time, the chair slouch places extreme amounts of strain on muscles and soft tissues. In return, this position is known to create lots of back, shoulder, and leg pain. It may seem like the natural and comfortable stance at first, but gradually being a chair sloucher will backfire on your health.

Solution: Proper Sitting Posture

To have good chair adequate you want to work at keeping all of your body parts aligned with the others. Always sit as far back as possible with your chair as close to the desk as possible (if you're sitting at one). Your feet should be flat on the ground, not crossed or shifted in any specific direction.

7 SIGNS YOU'LL NOTICE WHEN YOU HAVE BAD POSTURE

You may only have some of them, you may even have all of them, but the signs of bad posture you have are clear for everyone to see…including you. If you know what to look for! These are the 7 most common signs of bad posture that you're likely to see in yourself, your friends or family so keep your eye out!

1. Forward head carriage

How far forward does your head poke? Forward head carriage is usually the most common sign of bad posture. With good posture you want to see the hole in your ear sit over the middle of your shoulder. The further forward your head goes the more pressure it puts on the muscles and joints through your neck which lead to structural changes in your body that cause pain.

2. Slumped Shoulders

Slumped or rolled shoulders are another obvious sign of poor posture. Slumped shoulders often occur due to extended periods of sitting especially when leaning forward and staring at a computer screen.

Besides the obvious sign of your shoulders not sitting backwards another thing to look for is how much your chest sticks out. The further forward your shoulders come the more it depresses your chest. This causes tightening of the muscles in your chest as well as your neck and weakness in the muscles that are meant to hold your shoulders back.

3. Hunch Back

Hunch back can sound a little extreme. Generally what you want to look for is an increase in the curve through your mid-back, usually between your shoulder blades. This is known as an increased kyphosis. If you're noticing an increase in this curve your more than likely going to see both forward head carriage and slumped shoulders as well since they usually come about before the curve in your mid back increases.

4. Anterior Pelvic Tilt (Duck Bottom)

With bad posture your pelvis can change in one of two ways. Anterior pelvic tilt refers to your pelvis tilting into a forward position.

This tilt increases the curve through your lower back leading to more stress being put on certain joints there. On top of this it will lead to tight muscles at the top of your thigh (hip flexors) and very tight muscles in the back of your thigh (hamstrings). You may also notice it causes your stomach and bottom to stick out more than they should.

You'll notice pelvic tilt in a standing position when you're looking at yourself from a side on view. You might not be able to see it yourself so ask a friend or family member to check for you. Then look at theirs. Chances are at least one of you will have anterior pelvic tilt. This tends to be seen a lot more in women so ladies stay on the look out!

5. Posterior Pelvic Tilt (Sway Back)

Posterior pelvic tilt moves your pelvis in a backwards position. This a lot more common in men! What you want to look out for is how your pelvis is positioned in relation to your upper body. Again the best way to see this is from a side on view. If you notice that your upper body sways backwards or sits behind your pelvis you may very well have posterior pelvic tilt.

This also leads to a lot of stress on the joints in your lower back and tightening of specific muscles around your back, legs and hips.

6. Shoulder Tilt/Hike

Have you ever looked at yourself in the mirror and noticed one shoulder was higher than the other? You'd be right in thinking it was a sign of bad posture. Shoulder tilt occurs very commonly especially in a society where you most likely tend to be more dominant to one side of your body.

Think about the little things you do. Which side do you carry your bag with, answer your phone with, even brush your teeth with….Maybe you just tend to lean to one side when you're sitting at your desk. The more you use one side of your body the more overactive the muscles on that side become (specifically the muscles that cause elevation of your shoulder). This leads to hiking or tilting of one shoulder more than the other!

7. Flat Feet

Flat feet are very often missed as a sign of poor posture. Flat feet refers to the collapsing of the arches in your foot and are a sign of bad posture because they alter the biomechanics throughout the rest of your body. Try to picture your body as an entire unit. Changes you get to one area will always lead to changes in another area. (Feet will change the knees, which will change the hips and cause pelvic tilt etc.

Changes to the arches in your feet can lead to increased pressure on the joints in your entire body and also lead to pain.

WHAT CAUSES BAD POSTURE?

Most people attribute, at least to some degree, their neck or back pain to poor posture. Not surprisingly, these folks often rush to try a host of possible fixes that may range from exercise, massage, and chiropractic to yoga, Pilates, holistic therapies and workstation redesign. A trip to the doctor's office is also included in the quest for good body posture — by some, at least —particularly if there's pain.

But many of these well-meaning, albeit scared people have only a vague understanding of what posture really is, what causes problems with it and what kinds of things may help them improve theirs.

Good Posture Defined

Good posture is a form of fitness in which the muscles of the body support the skeleton in an alignment that is stable as well as efficient. This state of being called good posture is present both in stillness and in movement.

Unfortunately, numerous factors one may encounter in life can get in the way of good posture. For more people than not, bad posture comes about by the day to day effect of gravity as it acts on our structure. Bad posture may be due to an injury, a disease or because of genetics — i.e., the things that for the most part, you can't control. A combination of these factors is also quite common.

Determining the underlying factors to less than ideal posture may help guide you when choosing medical or holistic treatment, or when making lifestyle changes. To that end, here are 7 possible reasons why you may have bad posture. Consult with your licensed health provider for a deeper dive into any of these.

1. Injury and Muscle Guarding

Back and Neck Injuries - What You Need to Know About Injuries to the Back and Neck

Thomas Troy

After an injury, nearby muscles tend to go into spasm as a way of protecting the vulnerable area. While muscle spasms can limit your movements and cause pain, they also help keep your injured part stable, as well as protected from further injury risk.

The problem is, muscles that stay in spasm tend to weaken over time. The resulting imbalance between muscles that guard an injury and those still working normally may lead to aberrations in body posture.

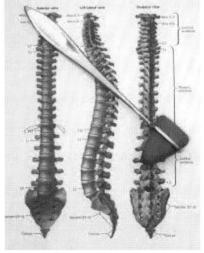

Muscles in spasm will likely work a diminished way, at least for a while after an injury, and usually, treatment in the form of massage and/or physical therapy will be needed to bring them back to optimal functioning.

2. Muscle Tension and Muscle Weakness

Similar to when you're injured, when the body has areas that are extra weak and/or strong, most likely, it will not be held upright against gravity in the most effective manner. This condition generally leads to poor posture and pain.

Excessive muscle strength and weakness may be brought about by a number of things, including the way you work out and the way you perform your routine tasks and chores.

3. Daily Habits Can Lead to Bad Posture

Your body will likely abandon good posture and alignment in order to find ways to accommodate muscle spasm, weakness, tension and/or imbalance between muscle groups.

This is because, in these cases, the body is forced to use alternate, but less efficient, patterns of muscle contraction and stretch. Called compensation, the body can still achieve its movement aim, but with comprised alignment.

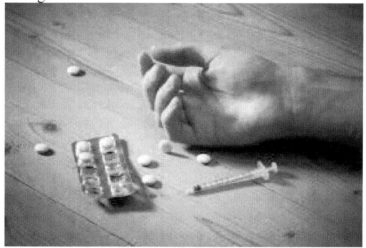

You might understand this process as a sort of detour. If you encounter an obstacle in the road while driving, you'd probably swerve to miss it but also to keep going towards your destination. The musculoskeletal system — in tandem with the nervous system — also develops detours to allow you to complete the intended movement even though some muscles and joints may not be contributing fully or working as part of the team.

4. Your Use of Technology and Your Posture

Your use of technology, whether you sit at a computer all day, use a tablet or cell phone or you work with several devices at once, can quickly take your body out of alignment. If you text incessantly, you may develop text neck, which is a condition in which your neck is held in too much flexion, or forward bending, for too long. This may lead to pain.

5. Mental Attitude and Stress May Lead to Bad Posture

Do you stress easily or have stressful relationships? If so, watch your posture!

Stress may lead to a decrease in full breathing as well as overly-contracted muscles, which in turn may compensate your ideal body posture.

6. Shoe Choice and The Way You Wear Them

Clothing, especially shoes, can affect posture.

Heels throw your body weight forward which can easily catapult you into misalignment.

And if you wear down either the outside or inside of the shoes faster — because of your usual weight-bearing habits — imbalanced kinetic forces will likely be translated up your ankle, knee, hip, and low back. This may lead to pain or bad posture in any of these joints, as well as your lumbar spine.

7. Heredity and Genetics

Sometimes it's just in the genes. For example, Scheuermann's Disease is a condition in which adolescent boys develop a pronounced kyphosis in their thoracic spines. Of course, in cases such as these, it's best to work with your doctor for treatment and management.

8. Types of Posture Problems

While all the above may cause or lead to bad posture, it's important to remember that for posture problems that are not medical or genetic in origin, four main types exist. These are the lordotic, kyphotic, flat and sway back types.

Each type has the capacity to disrupt good posture.

A 2018 study published in the March issue of Scoliosis Spinal Disorders points out that not only does muscle tension, strength and flexibility matter to the condition of your posture, but the degree to which muscles are used and exercise, as well.

12 EXERCISES TO IMPROVE YOUR POSTURE

- Child's pose
- Forward fold
- Cat cow
- Standing cat cow
- Chest opener
- High plank
- Side plank
- Downward-facing dog
- Pigeon pose
- Thoracic spine rotation
- Glute squeezes
- Isometric rows

Why posture's so important

Having good posture is about more than looking good. It helps you to develop strength, flexibility, and balance in your body. These can all lead to less muscle pain and more energy throughout the day. Proper posture also reduces stress on your muscles and ligaments, which can reduce your risk of injury.

Improving your posture also helps you become more aware of your muscles, making it easier to correct your own posture. As you work on your posture and become more aware of your body, you might even notice some imbalances or areas of tightness you weren't previously aware of.

Read on to learn how to do 12 exercises that'll help you stand a little taller.

1. Child's pose

This resting pose stretches and lengthens your spine, glutes, and hamstrings. The child's pose helps to release tension in your lower back and neck.

To do this:

Sit on your shinbones with your knees together, your big toes touching, and your heels splayed out to the side.

Fold forward at your hips and walk your hands out in front of you.

Sink your hips back down toward your feet. If your thighs won't go all the way down, place a pillow or folded blanket under them for support.

Gently place your forehead on the floor or turn your head to one side.

Keep your arms extended or rest them along your body.

Breathe deeply into the back of your rib cage and waist.

Relax in this pose for up to 5 minutes while continuing to breathe deeply.

2. Forward fold

This standing stretch releases tension in your spine, hamstrings, and glutes. It also stretches your hips and legs. While doing this stretch, you should feel the entire back side of your body opening up and lengthening.

To do this:

Stand with your big toes touching and your heels slightly apart.

Bring your hands to your hips and fold forward at your hips.

Release your hands toward the floor or place them on a block. Don't worry if your hands don't touch the ground — just go as far as you can.

Bend your knees slightly, soften your hips joints, and allow your spine to lengthen.

Tuck your chin into your chest and allow your head to fall heavy to the floor.

Remain in this pose for up to 1 minute.

3. Cat cow

Practicing cat cow stretches and massages your spine. It also helps to relieve tension in your torso, shoulders, and neck while promoting blood circulation.

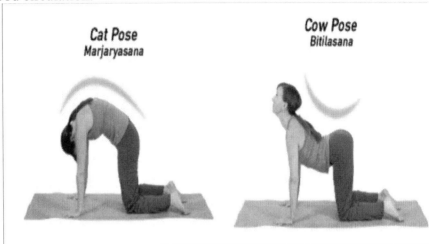

Cat Pose
Marjaryasana

Cow Pose
Bitilasana

To do this:

Come onto your hands and knees with your weight balanced evenly between all four points.

Inhale to look up, dropping your abdomen down toward the ground as you extend your spine.

Exhale and arch your spine toward the ceiling and tuck your chin into your chest.

Continue this movement for at least 1 minute.

4. Standing cat cow

Doing the cat cow stretch while standing helps to loosen up tightness in your back, hips, and glutes.

To do this:

Stand with your feet about hip-width apart with a slight bend in your knees.

Extend your hands in front of you or place them on your thighs.

Lengthen your neck, bring your chin toward your chest, and round your spine.

Then look up, lift your chest, and move your spine in the opposite direction.

Hold each position for 5 breaths at a time.

Continue this movement for a few minutes.

5. Chest opener

This exercise allows you to open and stretch your chest. This is especially useful if you spend most of your day sitting, which tends to make your chest move inward. Strengthening your chest also helps you stand up straighter.

To do this:

Stand with your feet about hip-width apart.

Bring your arms behind you and interlace your fingers with your palms pressing together. Grasp a towel if your hands don't reach each other.

Keep your head, neck, and spine in one line as you gaze straight ahead.

Inhale as you lift your chest toward the ceiling and bring your hands toward the floor.

Breathe deeply as you hold this pose for 5 breaths.

Release and relax for a few breaths.

Repeat at least 10 times.

Ready to see how this all fits into an exercise plan? Check out our guide for better posture in 30 days.

6. High plank

The high plank pose helps to relieve pain and stiffness throughout your body while strengthening your shoulders, glutes, and hamstrings. It also helps you develop balance and strength in your core and back, both important for good posture.

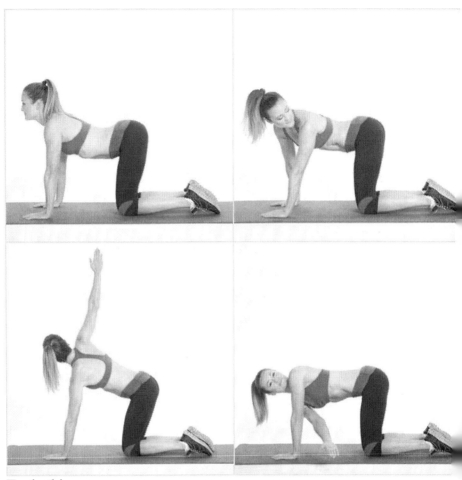

To do this:

Come onto all fours and straighten your legs, lift your heels, and raise your hips.

Straighten your back and engage your abdominal, arm, and leg muscles.

Lengthen the back of your neck, soften your throat, and look down at the floor.

Make sure to keep your chest open and your shoulders back.

Hold this position for up to 1 minute at a time.

7. Side plank

You can use a side plank to maintain the neutral alignment of your spine and legs. This energizing pose works the muscles in your sides and glutes. Strengthening and aligning these muscles helps to support your back and improve posture.

To do this:
From a high plank position, bring your left hand slightly in to center.
Shift your weight onto your left hand, stack your ankles, and lift your hips.
Place your right hand on your hip or extend it up toward the ceiling.
You can drop your left knee down to the floor for extra support.
Engage your abdominals, side body, and glutes as you maintain this pose.
Align your body in a straight line from the crown of your head to your heels.
Look straight ahead of you or up toward your hand.
Hold this pose for up to 30 seconds.
Repeat on the opposite side.

8. Downward-facing dog
This is a forward bend that can be used as a resting pose to balance out your body. The downward-facing dog pose helps to relieve back pain, while also strengthening and aligning your back muscles. Practicing it regularly helps to improve posture.
To do this:
Lying with your stomach on the floor, press into your hands as you tuck your toes under your feet and lift your heels.
Lift your knees and hips to bring your sitting bones up toward the ceiling.
Bend your knees slightly and lengthen your spine.
Keep your ears in line with your upper arms or tuck your chin all the way into your chest.
Press firmly into your hands and keep your heels slightly lifted.
Remain in this pose for up to 1 minute.

Have medical questions? Connect with a board-certified, experienced doctor online or by phone. Pediatricians and other specialists available 24/7.

9. Pigeon pose
This is a hip opener that also loosens up your spine, hamstrings, and glutes. The pigeon pose can also help to stretch your sciatic nerve and quadriceps. Opening and stretching these places in your body makes it easier to correct imbalances in your posture.

To do this:
Come down on all fours with your knees below your hips and your hands a little bit in front of your shoulders.
Bend your right knee and place it behind your right wrist with your right foot angled out to the left.
Rest the outside of your right shin on the floor.
Slide your left leg back, straighten your knee, and rest your thigh on the floor.
Make sure your left leg extends straight back (and not to the side).
Slowly lower your torso down to rest on your inner right thigh with your arms extended in front of you.
Hold this position for up to 1 minute.
Slowly release the position by walking your hands back toward your hips and lifting your torso.
Repeat on the left side.

10. Thoracic spine rotation
This exercise relieves tightness and pain in your back while increasing stability and mobility.
To do this:
Come onto all fours and sink your hips back down to your heels and rest on your shins.
Place your left hand behind your head with your elbow extended to the side.
Keep your right hand under your shoulder or bring it to center and rest on your forearm.

Exhale as you rotate your left elbow up toward the ceiling and stretch the front of your torso.

Take one long inhale and exhale in this position.

Release back down to the original position.

Repeat this movement 5 to 10 times.

Repeat on the opposite side.

11. Glute squeezes

This exercise helps to strengthen and activate your glutes while relieving lower back pain. It also improves the functioning and alignment of your hips and pelvis, leading to better posture.

To do this:

Lie on your back with your knees bent and your feet about hip-distance apart.

Keep your feet about a foot away from your hips.

Rest your arms alongside your body with your palms facing down.

Exhale as you bring your feet closer to your hips.

Hold this position for 10 seconds and then move them further away from your hips.

Continue this movement for 1 minute.

Do this exercise a few times per day.

12. Isometric rows

This exercise helps to relieve pain and stiffness from sitting in one place for too long. Isometric pulls work your shoulder, arm, and back muscles, giving you the strength to maintain good posture.

To do this:

Sit in a chair with a soft back.

Bend your arms so your fingers are facing forward and your palms are facing each other.

Exhale as you draw your elbows back into the chair behind you and squeeze your shoulder blades together.

Breathe deeply as you hold this position for 10 seconds.

On an inhale, slowly release to the starting position.

Repeat this movement for 1 minute.

Do this exercise several times throughout the day.

10-MINUTE WORKOUT TO FIX BAD POSTURE

In case you don't already know, there's a lot of value in having good posture. Not only does good posture boost your body image and make you look better in a suit, but it also helps decrease your likelihood of injury. It minimizes the load on your skeletal muscles, and enables your body to move more freely and efficiently. Poor posture can lead to anything from headaches, to rotator cuff injuries, back pain, and many other common ailments. In other words, fixing your posture could fix a lot of your problems.

Often times, when I help people feel what good posture actually is, the first thing they tell me is "I feel weird". This is because our bodies become used to the posture that we spend most of our time in. But this doesn't make your bad posture ok.

A quick exercise you can try at home is to balance something on your head – you'll probably straighten your spine and naturally place your head in a more correct position. The challenge then becomes to maintain this optimal posture throughout the majority of your day.

Which Muscles To Stretch vs. Strengthen?

If you search online, you'll find a seemingly unending list of exercises to do to improve your posture. All the information can get overwhelming, leaving you unsure of where to start. Let's simplify things bit.

There are a lot of common patterns of poor posture that people share – for example, forward head posture, forward rounded shoulders, and Janda's upper and lower crossed syndromes. These patterns frequently lead to specific muscles either being tight, or overstretched and weak.

Muscles to Stretch

If you had all day, the most common muscles that you should stretch include:
1. Suboccipitals
2. Pecs
3. Hip Flexors
4. Hamstrings

Muscles to Strengthen
And these are the most common muscles that you should strengthen:
1. Mid- and Lower-Trapezius
2. Anterior & Posterior Core
3. Glute Muscles

Depending on which specific postural pattern you tend to have, you may not need to stretch and strengthen all of the above, but I've also never seen people who are too flexible with the first list, or too strong with the second.

Ideally, your posture will match the alignment chart you see in the doctor's office.

When looking at the side, the plumb line (vertical line with your center of mass) should go through your ear and stay in line with the middle of your shoulder, middle of your pelvis, and down to the front of your heel (middle of the foot).

If you stand with your back to the wall, your head should be near the wall or touching when you look straight ahead (and not up). Your shoulders should rest near the wall with your thumbs pointing forward. You should have a small arch in your low back with your glutes touching the wall.

With some mindfulness of how you sit and stand in your daily life, you'll start to reinforce proper posture as a habit. If you want to kickstart the effects, here's an effective and efficient workout to reinforce good form and posture.

Workout (& Exercises) to Fix Poor Posture

The following exercises don't specifically target each and every muscle listed above, but instead aim to correct multiple muscles and body regions simultaneously for a more efficient workout.

Warm-up: Start by foam rolling your thoracic spine for 1-minute. This exercise helps straighten the upper spine. Since most of us tend to slouch more than we should, it's a good idea to start your workout with this.

Exercise Sets & Reps/Time

1. Wall Angels 2 x 10 reps (per min)
2. Hip Hinge with Hands Overhead 10 x 10 sec holds
3. Standing Horizontal Abduction with TRX (or Band) 10 x 10 sec holds
4. Farmer's Carry 2 x 1 min
5. Double- or Single-Leg Bridge Hold 2 x 1 min

Exercise Instructions:

1. Wall Angels

Instructions: Stand next to the wall, keep good posture, and raise your arms up the wall while keeping your core tight and ribcage down. Your spine should remain neutral, even as your raise your arms up. You should be able to extend your arms fully overhead while still touching the wall, without arching your back. If performed correctly, you'll feel the middle of your back and your abs contract to stabilize your spine.

2. Hip Hinge with Hands Over Head

Instructions: The emphasis here is on movement and flexibility. Performing the hip hinge with your arms overhead will stretch out your thoracolumbar fascia in the mid-back while challenging your core. The cues I constantly repeat for this exercise are, "Hips back, and hands high!"

3. Standing Horizontal Abduction with TRX (or Band)

The goal here is to strengthen your mid-back and shoulder blade muscles by opening up your chest and squeezing your shoulder blades together. Make sure not to flare your ribs out. Keep your core tight the entire time. You can perform this exercise with a resistance band, or a suspension trainer like the TRX. Stand tall and keep your head and neck in a straight line throughout the entire movement.

4. Farmer's Carry

Instructions: This exercise may actually be the most important. I mentioned earlier that most people will self-correct their posture if you put something on their head. The same thing happens when you carry something heavy. Carrying heavy things with bad posture is uncomfortable, and you won't be able to do it for long.

Do a farmer's carry with a heavy weight, focusing on standing tall, keeping your shoulders back, and minimizing any spinal movement. This exercise teaches you just how tall you can be, and need to be when lifting heavy weights. Remember this feeling as you go through all of your other exercises.

For an extra challenge (only if you have the adequate flexibility), try a waiter's carry, holding the kettlebell in the overhead position.

5. Double- or Single-Leg Bridge Hold

Instructions: Finish your posture-fixing workout by challenging your posterior muscles. Progress to the single-leg bridge once you've built up your strength and endurance. Not only will this exercise improve the endurance of your back muscles, but you'll also strengthen your glutes.

If you mix this workout into your routine 2-3 days per week, you should definitely see improvements in your posture. But the goal is to have this carry over into your daily life – when you sit at your desk, when you're standing and talking to people, and in your other workouts.

MORE EXERCISES THAT CAN FIX BAD POSTURE

Our posture is directly affected by the condition of the spine. The mobility of the spine in a healthy, trained person is unique! It can turn over its entire length by as much as 180 degrees in any direction — and such abilities are absolutely independent of age. Therefore, in order to have a truly royal posture, you need to know how to perform exercises aimed at stretching the spine and the entire back as a whole.

To feel correct posture, stand up straight, feet shoulder-width apart, inhale with a full chest, and spread your shoulders while simultaneously pulling the shoulder blades together and pulling your shoulders back and forth a little. Put the chest forward with the coccyx looking down. The top of the head is stretched upwards.

For most people, this way of standing will not only be uncomfortable, but it will also be quite hard to maintain. Fortunately, the sooner you begin to perform exercises that straighten the spine, the faster you will correct your posture and the more athletic your figure will become.

Exercises to get better posture

This is a list of simple exercises that straighten the spine and improve posture. Do them for 20 minutes, 3 times a week and you will quickly notice positive results including reduced back pain and less overall fatigue.

1. Baby pose

This exercise is also used for relaxation. Get in this position by sitting on the heels, your big toes touching each other, and the knees diluted. When you exhale, slowly lower the body down, then pull your arms forward. Breathe quietly. Try to pull the coccyx back and forth, directing the chest down to the floor.

2. Cat stretching

This exercise is used to improve the mobility of the spine. The starting position requires you to be on all fours. While inhaling, strain the press, then bend the back, pulling the head as high as possible and pulling the coccyx back and up. When you exhale, round the spine as hard as possible, aiming your head down.

3. The bending tree pose

This exercise is great for your balance development. The starting position is standing, legs slightly shoulder-width apart, coccyx pointing down. Upon inhalation, raise your hands upward, pulling your fingers into a lock. As you exhale, slowly feel the sensation of your muscles in the body as you bend without changing the position of the thighs. Hold for 10-20 seconds.

4. Balancing table pose

This exercise is designed to strengthen the hull and balance development. The starting position is on all fours. Upon inhalation, take the right leg back, straighten it, then pull your left arm forward. Strain the press and try to keep a straight line. Hold for 10-20 seconds, then change your hand.

5. Pose of traction

This exercise is for stretching the spine. The starting position is standing up. Upon exhalation, slowly and with a sense of control, lower the body down, dragging your head to the floor. Slightly point the hips upwards and straighten the knees without straining your neck. Take 5-7 slow, deep breaths, then gently return to the vertical position.

6. Scroll lying down

This exercise is for stretching the spine. The starting position has you lying on your back, hands spread apart, palms down. Bend your legs at the knee and pull them up. Upon exhalation, gently push your palms on the knees, trying to lower them further to your side.

7. Dynamic plank

This exercise is great for stretching the spine. Begin the exercise in the plank position with the body stretched out in a straight line. When you exhale, direct the buttocks upward, making sure that the press is tense and the lower back is kept straight (this is much more important than the bent knees). Hold for 10-20 seconds.

Features and contraindications

Exercises to improve posture are always performed neatly, slowly and with full movement control. If you're not able to get into a certain position, do not try to force your body with effort or pressure. If there is a sharp pain, stop the workout immediately.

If in the gym you work with dumbbells, it's important to distribute the weight evenly — in other words, there should be an equivalent weight in each hand. Don't lean back. The back should be straightened. If you follow these rules when working with dumbbells, your back will become strengthened rather than suffer.

WAYS TO FIX YOUR TERRIBLE POSTURE

Good posture isn't just about looks. How we sit, stand, and walk affect both our health and our moods. So, stop slouching and get centered with these top 10 posture tips.

1. Get the Wii Fit

This isn't an option for everyone, since it involves investing in an expensive video game system, but if you have the Nintendo Wii or Wii U, I highly recommend the Wii Fit. Sometimes you can find the game, balance board, and fitness tracker for just $20—well worth the price for a unique game that focuses on measuring your balance and keeping you moving every day. In the first week of playing the game, my posture went from severely unbalanced to the right to centered (and I think about my posture constantly now, which I guess is a good thing). If you don't have the Wii or Wii U, perhaps play any other video games standing up. Sitting all day is killing us and many of us could be better off standing more.

2. Test Your Posture and Learn to Stand Properly

That all depends, of course, if you're standing properly to begin with. Test your back and neck posture against a wall or check this illustration to find any areas you need to work on when standing. Become more aware of your feet when you're standing and adjust your weight so it's distributed evenly across both feet. These seven moves will test your basic mobility and core strength.

3. Do Yoga or Work on Your Core Strength

Exercises that strengthen your core will help you stand taller and help you maintain the proper posture. I like yoga because it also emphasizes body awareness and balance—and you can work up to some pretty badass poses. Pilates and any other exercises that focus on your core will help with your posture too.

4. Sit at a 135 Degree Angle

When you do have to sit, make sure you've got a good chair that supports your back and is ergonomic for your workspace (more on that below). Sitting at a 135-degree angle could put less strain on your spine, but you'd have to adjust your workspace accordingly. If you don't care to recline, check out this animated guide to the do's and don'ts of sitting.

5. Adjust Your Posture in Every Situation

It's not just at our desks that we have to think about our posture. We need to sit up straight when driving (adjusting your rear view mirror could help). Our posture when we're sleeping, the type of pillow we use, and the type of mattress we sleep on will affect how we hold ourselves during the day. If you have to work from bed, do it in a way that won't wreck your posture. And in the kitchen, you might need to adjust the height of your counters to keep from hunching over.

6. Learn to Breathe Properly

How we breathe can deeply affect how we move and how we feel. Learn to breathe more effectively, using your diaphragm, and try breathing exercises that focus on lengthening your spine and engaging your waist muscles and lower core muscles.

7. Use Apps to Improve Your Posture

Remembering to stand and sit properly is hard work, so thankfully there are apps to help us out. Nekoze is a cute app that uses your Mac's camera to keep an eye on your posture—a cat (icon) will warn you when you're slouching. There are other posture trainers for iOS and Android, but if you're not into apps using your camera, build your own posture sensor for your chair.

8. Hold Your Phone and Tablet Properly

Constantly craning your neck down to stare at our phones isn't helping. Try holding your phone straight in front of you instead of bending your head down, and similarly propping your tablet up perpendicular to the table if you're just reading.

9. Fix Your Workstation

If you're a desk jockey, you might get the most posture improvement from setting up your workstation properly. Figure out the ideal desk height, whether sitting or standing, and keep your feet flat on the floor when sitting (an easy way to find the right seat high is to level it with your knees). Here's our complete guide to setting up an ergonomic workspace.

10. Do Posture-Correcting Exercises

Good posture involves training your body to be in the proper position, with the least amount of strain possible on your supporting muscles. In addition to these do's and don'ts for posture, we've shared several simple exercises you can do to improve your posture.

WAYS TO IMPROVE BACK PAIN

Should you wear a back brace and take it easy? Maybe not.

Like the nearly 80% of Americans who will experience a back problem during their lifetime, Beverly Hayes suffers from back pain. For many, the injury is triggered by a strenuous activity, like gardening or weight lifting. Others simply bend down to pick up a pencil and their back gives out.

"It felt like a screwdriver was piercing through my bones," the 46-year-old Chicago artist says about the pain that developed shortly after she ran a half-marathon. "It took over my life. I couldn't bend down or sleep — I was petrified I would never feel normal again."

Mary Ann Wilmarth, DPT, a spokeswoman for the American Physical Therapy Association and chief of physical therapy at Harvard University, says it is critical that people address any back pain or injury right away. "Early intervention can help prevent a chronic problem from developing and obviate the need for medication and surgery," she says.

Thanks to a combination of activity, core strengthening exercises, and physical therapy, Hayes says her symptoms have improved dramatically over the last year. Here are 12 ways to help alleviate back pain:

1. Limit Bed Rest

Studies show that people with short-term low-back pain who rest feel more pain and have a harder time with daily tasks than those who stay active.

"Patients should avoid more than three days of bed rest," says Mike Flippin, MD, an orthopaedic surgeon who specializes in back and spine care at San Diego Medical Center. "I encourage my patients to get moving as quickly as possible."

2. Keep Exercising

Activity is often the best medicine for back pain. "Simple exercises like walking can be very helpful," Wilmarth says. "It gets people out of a sitting posture and puts the body in a neutral, upright position."

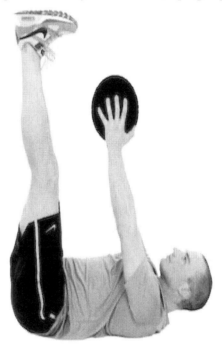

But remember to move in moderation, Flippin says. "Stay away from strenuous activities like gardening and avoid whatever motion caused the pain in the first place."

3. Maintain Good Posture

The pain may have started after a long workout at the gym, but the strain that caused it has probably been building for years. Wilmarth says most people have poor posture when going about their daily activities, putting unnecessary strain on their backs.

"Little things add up," she says. "You can increase the pressure on your back by 50% simply by leaning over the sink incorrectly to brush your teeth. Keeping the right amount of curvature in the back takes pressure off the nerves and will reduce back pain."

4. See a Specialist

Developing an individualized exercise plan is essential to managing chronic back pain, says D. Scott Davis, PT, MS, EdD, OCS, an orthopaedic physical therapist and associate professor at West Virginia University.

"There is no magic aspirin that addresses lower back pain in everyone," Davis says. "Some patients need more core strengthening while others benefit mainly from stretching and improving flexibility. Find a physical therapist, exercise physiologist, or chiropractor who specializes in back care. They will match you with the right exercise plan."

5. Strengthen Your Core

Most people with chronic back pain would benefit from stronger abdominal muscles.

"The torso is a combination of many muscle groups working together," Frank B. Wyatt, EdD, professor of exercise physiology at Missouri Western State University, tells WebMD in an email. "If the abdominals are weak, other areas must pick up the slack. When we strengthen the abdominals, it often reduces the strain on the lower back."

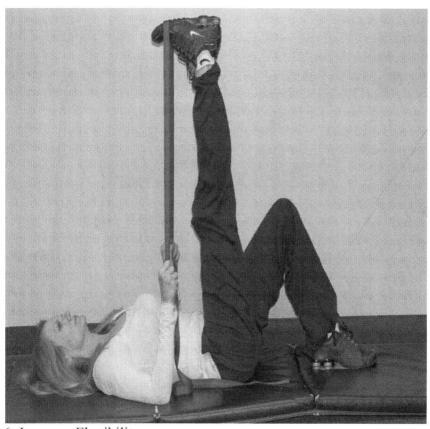

6. Improve Flexibility

Too much tension and tightness can cause back pain. "Our goal in increasing flexibility is to put an equal load throughout the body from the feet all the way up to the head," Davis says. "One good exercise is to sit on the edge of the bed with one leg extended and the other one on the floor. Give your hamstrings a stretch by leaning forward while keeping your back in a neutral position."

7. Ditch the Brace

It's tempting to baby your back muscles, but Davis says braces should be used sparingly. "Braces are helpful for strenuous activities, like heavy lifting, but only keep them on for 15 minutes at a time," he says. If you wear a brace all day, the muscles — which should be providing stability — weaken and you will have less core strength.

8. Apply Ice and Heat

Heating pads and cold packs can comfort tender trunks. Most doctors recommend using ice for the first 48 hours after an injury -- particularly if there is swelling — and then switching to heat.

But "it is difficult to say if ice or heat is more beneficial," Flippin says. "I recommend that patients use whichever they find comforting as long as their skin is protected."

9. Sleep the Right Way

The amount of rest you get is important, and so is the position you get it in. "Sleeping in a bad position or on a mattress without support can cause back pain," Wilmarth says.

Some pointers:

Back sleepers should put pillows under their knees.

Side sleepers should place pillows between their knees to keep their spine in a neutral position.

Stomach sleeping causes the neck and head to twist and can put undue stress on the back.

10. Quit Smoking

Lighting up doesn't just damage your lungs; it can also hurt your back.

A study recently published in the American Journal of Medicine found that current and former smokers are more likely to have back pain when compared with people who have never smoked.

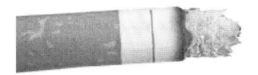

"Nicotine causes the small blood vessels to constrict and decreases the delivery of blood to the soft tissue," Flippin says. "I tell all my patients that quitting smoking could help alleviate their back pain."

11. Try Talk Therapy

Back pain is often seen with issues such as depression and anxiety, says Alex Moroz, MD, associate professor of rehabilitation medicine at NYU Langone Medical Center.

"Your emotional state colors the perception of pain," Moroz says. "Therapy can be a helpful part of rehabilitation."

12. Use Relaxation Techniques

Research shows that practices such as meditation, deep breathing, tai chi, and yoga, which help put the mind at rest, can do wonders for the back.

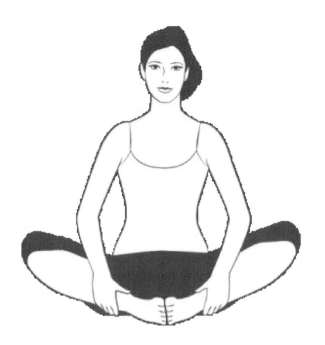

BETTER POSTURE MEANS SITTING AT THE OFFICE PROPERLY ON AN ALIGNED PELVIS.

Before discussing how to improve sitting at the office, let's first begin by talking about what we are sitting on. Your pelvis consists of several bones. You have your two large hip bones, or your ilium bones. The lower part of the iliums are your ischiums which are your sitting bones. The sacrum is an important bone, considered by past cultures as a "sacred" bone, hence the name. It is found where the base of your spine or vertebra meet the pelvis. Let's not forget the coccyx, the tailbone. This is the affected anatomy of the pelvis, at least the bones anyway. Now let's talk how we are putting our pelvis to use while we are sitting at the office (or school, or home). Perhaps a modified stooping position would be a better way to sit at the office. There is a difference between sitting and stooping. One is more likely lead to a better posture and possibly make you feel better, even as you are sitting at the office.

When we sit at the office we mimic what has been done for centuries. In some parts of the world, stooping rather than sitting is the normal way to rest for short periods of time. Quite often, because they stoop, the people of these countries maintain a desirable posture. I suggest that we all consider a modified stooping position rather than a typical sitting position. I won't suggest that you go to your office and throw out your chair and stoop before your computer to begin the day (come to think of it, maybe that's an idea). Let's learn more about properly sitting at the office.

Allow me to suggest the following way to stoop rather than sit, both at the office and at home. You will find as you assume a stooping position that your back, legs, pelvis, their ligaments, joints, and backbones are stretched nearly to their apex. That's to say they are stretched very well. This stretching is a good way to acquire a nice posture. You can assume this posture while sitting at the office and I'll discuss just how.

1. When sitting at the office correctly, choose a chair built low to the ground but with a high back to rest your spine. (Unfortunately high backed chairs are hard to find). Choose one where the seat will be approximately 18 inches from the ground. It is desired that your knees are above your hips. This position of the knees helps to acquire a good posture while sitting at the office.

2. If your chair seat is higher than two feet from the floor, use a footstool. Again, while sitting at the office, the object is to position your knees to be slightly above your hips. This lengthens the thigh muscles and reduces fat buildup on the buttocks. Lengthening the leg muscles helps to gain a pleasing posture.

3. Adopt a sitting posture at the office that helps you look, feel, and perform better. Lean a little forward and raise your chin just a little. A lowered, modified stooping position allows for a better sitting posture to take place, and your eyes are more level to the computer screen (great for a balanced head position). A modified stooped seating position encourages your head and neck to be positioned more aligned with the spine (and helps to remove a double chin and a "too forward" head position). Who knew that sitting at the office properly would have so many advantages.

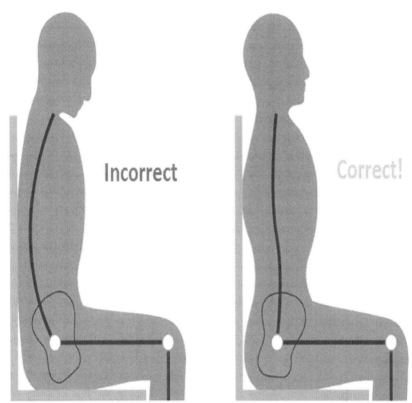

Incorrect

Correct!

To gain poise while sitting at the office it is best that your head pivots and balances upon the uppermost disk of your spine. Balance and turn your head at the C1 disk, and not the C7 disk found at the top of the shoulders.

While sitting at a modified stooping position, one's chest rises during this sitting adaptation. What this position is doing is straightening the back, raising the shoulders, and enabling you to sit in a more balanced upper body posture. We are removing the excessive curve from our lower back and relieving the pressure on our sacrum and pelvis. We are adjusting a tilted pelvis so that it is more perpendicular to the ground. We are thus correctly sitting on our ischiums, our sitting bones.

Any time we can lighten our load we do it, especially at the sacrum, this sensitive location of our body. A note of important information is that the small of the back is the nerve center of our body. Impulses are sent to and from our extremities, small of the back, and brain at super quick speeds. We want no impedance at this "junction box", the small of the back. Let's continue to learn how to improve our posture by sitting well at the office.

4. Once seated in this more stooped position, take a moment to enjoy the adjustment to your body and posture. Notice the feel of the upward push of your upper body from your properly positioned pelvis. Note that your sacrum bone is centered, and is now a proper, strong base for your spine. Also your entire, more aligned spine pushes your head higher. Yes it is possible to sit at the office and improve your posture.

Overall you've acquired a better posture and are enjoying a more better seating position while sitting at the office. Let's talk about the physiology of our body when sitting. This will help you understand what happens as we improve our posture and you change for the better. When lengthening the spine and balancing the head atop a free and more aligned, vertical neck, the shoulders are pulled up by the muscles attached to the clavicles, scapula and sternum. These muscles are attached to your skull and are doing the job of suspending the shoulders at a higher position. A parallel would be like the ropes from the mast of a sailing ship that hold up the yardarms (your shoulders). These ropes raise the sails so they can capture the wind. We're getting a little off topic but this is great to know. Free your neck muscles and neck bones. Align your cervical bones (neck bones) with your entire spine. Again, insure the head is positioned and balanced above the shoulders so that it, and you, have grace and poise. Loosen you jaw. Remember to turn your head at the C1 vertebra of your spine. Breath easily as your more open chest cavity accepts more air like the sails of a sailing vessel. Doing this while sitting at the office will bring about good posture and will likely improve life at the office.

5. Perhaps while sitting at the office, and at home, you use a "physio ball to gain good posture." This air filled exercise ball comes in various sizes and they are not expensive. When you sit on one, you are generally

positioned so that your bottom is lower than your knees. Be prepared for a workout when using this ball. Talk about a passive exercise. Not! If you have any twist or turn in your pelvis, the ball will duly note this. If your iliums are rotated this could mean you have an upslip or downslip where the sacrum meet the iliums. The sacrum could be rotated as well. This puts a stress on the iliums and the spine and overall. The muscles of your back, butt, and legs will have to adjust properly so that the pain you may feel from your muscle imbalance can be alleviated. Using the physio ball you'll be engaging muscles that you should have been using all along for a good posture. There is some pain when replacing the muscles you were using improperly, while you had poor posture. Your old way of using the wrong muscles won't be at all happy when you adjust your way of sitting at the office. Your proper muscles that you are using to sit are now literally fighting against the improper muscles that you've used previously. In other words, you are inhibiting your old habits and old habits die hard.

Did I say this was going to be easy? However, within months or a year or so it will become easier. Your pelvis will become more aligned and sitting at the office will be more enjoyable, at least much less painful. After practicing these better sitting techniques, you will know how to move and adjust your body to attain the posture you desire.

Lengthening and stretching your body is key, and you can make these stretches, subtly while sitting at the office. Soon your adjusted body won't permit you to slouch and cause your muscles to do the wrong thing. Your muscles will react like those muscles of people with grace and poise. Your muscles, like theirs, will want to be used efficiently. Later your muscles, when used improperly, will tell you when you are holding your body asymmetrical or moving improperly and unbalanced. Sitting at the office will be much more enjoyable. Of course work may not change, but I am not going to go there.

Now or soon enough, enduring the painful joints and muscles of a poor posture will occur less often. Your muscles that grow accustomed to holding up a more aligned spine and body will tell you when you are not holding your posture in an upright position. It will be painful when you assume a bad posture, when you are too quick and unsteady in your movements. Instead you'll take the time to move more gracefully. You'll use your body efficiently to take you from one place to another. You'll like what you see in your newly acquired posture, and others will too. This is an experience that I assure you will be a great time in your life. Doors will open and birds will take to the skies all from learning to sit properly at the office.

POSTURE AND NECK PAIN - IMPROVE IT TO GET RID OF IT

Posture and Pain

As much as it pains me to say it, mom was right about posture. Slouching contributes to many people's headaches, neck pain, and back pain. The body is designed to sit and stand up straight. If you are standing with good posture there is much less strain on muscles, tendons, and joints compared to slouching. The body was not designed to sit with a rounded back and shoulders, or with the head leaning forward. This position may feel comfortable but several muscles are working overtime.

Have you ever held a 7 pound bowling ball? Did you hold it close to your chest or out in front of you? How heavy does that bowling ball feel when your arms are extended straight? Can you hold that position for a minute? Most people's arms will begin shaking and burning within 30 seconds. The muscles are working very hard to hold the ball up in the air. However, you could hold the ball for 30 minutes if it was positioned closer to your chest. The muscles are not working near as hard the closer the ball is to your center of gravity.

Slouching Matters

Not many people are interested in the physics. I'm sure we could calculate and compare the amount of energy required to hold the ball 5 minutes at arms length verses your chest. The difference in Newtons (measuring unit of forces) would be significant, and at the same time conceptually meaningless. (I'm sure one of my engineering patients will send me the correct answer with a simplified explanation. There is a lunch reward for the first one to do so.

I cannot conceptualize the effort required for 3,000 Newtons. But I do know that I hold things closer to my body whenever possible. Why should I spend the energy to do it the hard way, and potentially hurt myself in the process?

Why Does Posture Matter

Slouching makes certain muscles work extra hard. That 7 pound bowling ball on top of your neck, also known as your head, is held up by muscles and joints. The spine is a series of bones that support your body weight. The spine has several curves that absorb the weight like a spring. Slouching straightens the spring and increases the forces at certain points of the spring, thereby increasing the effort to keep you upright.

If you sit at a computer with perfect posture the curves of your spine would absorb most of the forces, and the muscles would evenly distribute the remaining work load. Ideally your ear is directly above your shoulder which is above your waist. Moving your head and shoulders forward two inches changes the curve in your neck and back to a less desirable position. Certain muscles are now working harder to support the structural change.

The increased effort does not seem like much; however, how long are you going to be sitting at the computer today? Multiply the increased effort by the amount of hours and days. Now we can see the small change makes a huge difference to the muscles weekly workload.

Taking this a step further, do you sit with great posture in the car, couch, or kitchen table? How much time in a day is spent slouching? Do you slouch more than two inches? Most people slouch through the entire day when sitting, and every inch dramatically increases the workload on the muscles.

Over the course of months and years, many people develop headaches, neck pain, or back pain as a result of poor posture. The muscles and joints have been overworked for years and have been gone through subtle signs of injury. After a while people begin to notice increased tightness and loss of flexibility in their neck, shoulder, and back muscles. They might begin to complain of muscle aches and soreness. People start asking for neck and back rubs because of muscle aches. "Knots" in the muscles begin to form and never go away.

Bad Posture has Been Causing You Pain

Looking backward, people realize an increased amount of stiffness and mild soreness in their neck and back. They begin to have more episodes of dull neck and back pain. The number of instances of sharp pain or twinges increases through the years. They begin having several days of moderate dull pain and very limited motion. The moderate back pain does go away after a few days but another episode occurs within a few months. They start waking up more often with "stiff necks."

People start to feel fatigued at the end of the day more often and can't wait for the weekend to recover. Some people start to have mild headaches at the end of the day, that then go away with a little rest or Advil. The headaches intensity, frequency, and duration is worse with increased stress or work hours. The subtle signs have been there for years, now is the time to correct the underlying problem.

Posture is a habit. It can be improved but it will take time and effort. As you begin sitting with good posture it will feel very uncomfortable, and you may feel soreness in new places. At first you might hold the position for 5 minutes before slouching again. Then it will increase to 10 minutes, and then to 20 before slouching. With sustained effort and awareness you will begin to have better posture throughout the whole day. Since good posture requires less muscle effort, within a few weeks you will feel a decrease in muscle soreness and fatigue.

Ways to Improve Posture at Home

I always suggest putting a sticky note on your computer monitor or work phone that says "Sit UP!" You will be amazed at how often you find yourself slouching. Some people will set a phone alarm or Outlook reminder for 20 minute intervals. Changing the habit requires effort and constant reminding at the beginning.

The quickest way to improve your posture is to play a game with your coworkers. Put a change jar on everyone's desk. If someone catches you slouching you owe them a quarter. It becomes a rewarding challenge to catch people slouching. It will probably cost $10 by lunchtime, but you will quickly find yourself sitting up straight with every squeak of a chair. In a cubical work setting, the top of heads begin to pop up straight like Prairie Dog Fields whenever a coworker starts talking.

Identify the times and places that you are slouching the worst, such as home computer, laptops, Ipads, driving, couches, standing, or walking. Focus on increasing the amount of time spent with better posture in each of these situations. Changing a habit will take time and effort but can be done with the right dedication.

7 FACTORS TO POOR POSTURE AND 2 STEPS YOU CAN TAKE RIGHT NOW TO BETTER YOUR OWN

Have you ever noticed a famous actor, known for their good looks, maybe Brad Pitt, standing stooped over? Of course not! Part of the appeal is their tall, proud posture, whether you consciously notice or not. Perhaps that's why no childhood is complete without an occasional reminder to "Sit up straight!" Your mom was training you to become a Hollywood star.

While the desire for your own good posture could be due to the effect that poor posture has on your visual appearance, it may surprise you that posture has much more to do with whether you look proper or sloppy. Let's look at another type of celebrity - a singer such as Adele, and try a little experiment on yourself. Sing your favourite song, or the national anthem with your shoulders rounded forward and head stooped down. Your whole chest caves in and prohibits your lungs from expanding and your voice from belting out those big musical notes. It's much harder to sing properly without good posture. Remember Usain Bolt, the fastest human? Do you think he'd run as fast and place as well if he kept his head down?

If you're concerned with your health you should know that the way you carry your body physically can have a major impact on your physical performance and mental sense of well-being. Studies are now showing the connection between poor posture and health problems ranging from weight gain, insomnia, and even depression and mental decline. Chiropractors are well aware of the significance of this connection between posture and health, which makes them a reliable authority on this and how it relics on good spinal health.

There are many causes of poor posture. In some people, unfortunately postural issues are due to other conditions or diseases that involve bone deformity or bone loss, however, in the vast majority of cases, posture is directly related to a person's habits and daily activities. Here are some of the most common causes of poor posture:

• Looking down a lot during activities such as using a cellphone or playing video games
• Working at a desk or computer for long periods of time (even at a desk with good ergonomics)
• Poor ergonomics at work (chairs, desks, keyboards)
• Improper sleep support (mattress, pillows)
• Obesity
• Muscles weakness
• Poor self-esteem (people with low self-esteem tend to have a flexed/inward posture as a way to avoid being noticed)

As noted, there can be other health conditions and diseases that can contribute to poor posture, but as you can see, most contributors to poor posture are also things that are within your control.

Chiropractors and other health experts have found that people who have a tendency to slouch while standing, sitting, and even walking also tend to experience many kinds of health conditions, which can be mild or even severe. Many health problems such as headaches, muscle stiffness, shortness of breath, susceptibility to infectious illnesses, may actually be indirectly impacted by your posture and the positioning of your spinal column.

Your spine is important because it keeps your entire body in alignment and balance. It also houses and is meant to protect your central nervous system (spinal cord and brain). Your nervous system is responsible for the communication between your body and brain. The better your spinal alignment, the easier it is for your brain and body to share information and maintain good posture. Slouching, and being in poor posture makes it harder for this to happen - signals don't transmit as well and muscles have to work harder to try to keep you upright. This extra, more difficult work can degrade the health of the spine and nervous system over time. When your brain and body need to work harder on your posture, they work less on keeping your other systems and functions working optimally. As this happens to the nervous system, other functions of the body may begin to have trouble working correctly, leading to inflammation, digestive issues, and more.

How To Keep Good Posture All Day Every Day

If you want to avoid these health problems, you'll want to focus on maintaining proper posture as often as you can. It may be as simple as reminding yourself throughout the day to keep your shoulders pulled back, your head held high atop your neck and torso, and your spine in a neutral position as much it can.

If you find it difficult to maintain these positions of proper posture, it is a sign you need the professional help of a chiropractor. Your poor posture can be due to a combination of factors that include poor spinal alignment, poor nervous system signal flow, and muscle weakness. In most cases, these problems can all be corrected with a properly designed and executed plan that addresses all three of these issues as needed.

Have someone take a picture of you standing without shoes on a flat surface, looking ahead of you. Think of a side profile of a police mug shot, for your whole body, top to bottom. The person will likely have to stand 10-15 feet away.

Draw a straight vertical line from the inside of your ear down to the floor. If the line doesn't pass through the middle of your shoulder, hip, knee and ankle, it's likely you have poor posture.

If you're unsure that you're assessing your posture picture correctly, enlist a friend or family member to do this with you.

Made in United States
Troutdale, OR
05/30/2024

20227538R00040